It's Okay to Ta~~ke~~ ~~estrogen~~ ...
estrogen may ~~be~~ ...

"What ~~c~~ ...
ed for tl ...
learned a lot! I found the book well organized, fast and
very easy reading. The information was presented factu-
ally, and objectively, yet with a great deal of sensitivity
and as a result the information was much easier to
'accept'. All the questions I had on the subject, and then
some, were answered very comprehensively. I will recommend this book to my nursing colleagues, my physician
and his colleagues and definitely to my female friends
young and 'old'. Actually, I believe it's a book most
women should read. I am now definitely a believer in
estrogen therapy, especially since all those myths and
misconceptions that I have been too remiss in researching
or asking my physician about have been eliminated."
— Gail P. Tiwanak, R.N., M.B.A., Project Director,
Clinical Information System, The Queen's Medical Center,
Honolulu, Hawaii

"This book is written in a flowing question and answer
style that is very easy to read. It takes you stepwise
from basic concepts about estrogen all the way to state
of the art therapy of the menopausal woman. 'It's Okay
to Take Estrogen' is an encyclopedic work that is invalu-
able for any woman trying to decide the issue of estrogen replacement therapy." — Morton Kousen, M.D.,
F.A.C.O.G., York, Pennsylvania

It's Okay To Take Estrogen

In fact, estrogen may be your best
friend for life!

C. Alan Sevener, M.D.

Eclectic Publishing, Inc.
Fresno, California

Published by:
Eclectic Publishing, Inc.
P.O. Box 28340
Fresno CA 93729-8340

Allen County Public Library
900 Webster Street
Box 2270
Fort Wayne, IN 46801-2270

Library of Congress Catalog Card Number: 94-61494

Publisher's Cataloging in Publication Data on page 111.

ISBN: 0-9642282-9-7

Printed in the United States of America.

Dedication...

In gratitude for their trust, their honesty, and their willingness to allow me to share in their care...

This book is lovingly dedicated to each of the thousands of women who have honored me over the years with that trust...

And to a better life for them and all women with whom I share this information.

Table of Contents

Preface 8

Introduction 10

What's happening to me? 13

A is for Attitude. 19

B is for Bones. 23

C is for Circulation. .27

Irregular Periods: Your early warning system. .29

Estrogen Replacement Therapy. 31

Alternative routes to the same end. 37

So... I have to take medicine? 41

How much is enough? 45

Do I have to have periods? 51

Please don't take my ovaries! 55

Some straight talk about sex. 59

What about cancer? .65

What about those package inserts? 71

Estrogen increases your safety. 79

Why haven't I heard any of this before? 83

Your future... your choice. 87

References 95

Preface

How well do you understand your body's hormone system? As a practicing Obstetrician/Gynecologist for over 20 years, I have discovered that most women have very little knowledge of this complex system, or the profound effect it has on virtually every aspect of their lives.

A routine office visit lasts only minutes. During that brief period of time, it is difficult for your health care professional to answer all the questions you might have about hormonal changes taking place in your body. Compounding this problem: studies show that in face-to-face communication, we remember only 30 percent of what we hear.

It is important for women to understand their hormone systems and the profound effect changes in their hormone levels can have upon their lives. Since this information is so often unavailable, I have written this book. While by no means a textbook on body chemistry, it does offer an easy-to-understand overview of your hormone system. It identifies signs and symptoms of specific hormone disorders, and explains why it is so vital to your continued well-being to address these problems.

This book presents that information in an easy-to-understand manner. It is designed to be a learning tool, as well as a handy reference on the subject of hormones and estrogen replacement therapy. I hope it helps cut through the confusion stemming from well-intentioned but misinformed sources—be they friends, family, sensationalized media reports, or even members of my own health care community.

Although the information presented is drawn from a variety of scientific and professional sources as well as my own clinical experience, this book is not intended to be the last (or only) word on the subject of hormones. It is certainly not intended to take the place of the one-on-one relationship you have with your own physician or other health professional. Nor is it intended to give specific professional advice in any specific instance. That advice must come from your own physician or other health professional.

I hope the information in this book will help you understand that advice, and enable you to be a better-informed and more confident participant in decision-making regarding your own health care.

C. Alan Sevener, M.D.

Introduction

My working title for this book was *"Those Confusing Hormones*, or *Why estrogen may be your best friend for the rest of your life."* Since you are reading this, I can assume you have an interest in the subject. And if you're confused about hormones, join the crowd!

I've spent the past 20 years discussing hormones with women, their family and friends, and fellow practitioners. In the course of those conversations, I've heard every question imaginable on the subject. Twenty years of researching answers to those questions has convinced me this is one of the most confusing subjects around!

Why are hormones so confusing? That's the purpose of this book: to explain where the confusion comes from, who is responsible, why it continues and what can be done to get rid of it.

If you are a person who thinks you may need hormones then this book is primarily for you!

If you have a loved one whom you think may need hormones, this book is also for you.

If you are a practitioner of the healing arts, this book is also for you. It will answer many of your questions. It will help you to be more aware of the immense benefit you can be to those who put their faith and trust in you. It will help you to guide them through a difficult time in their lives and on to a better life ahead.

"Why is this book any different than the tons of others out there that talk about hormones? "

This book has only one purpose: to make hormones easy to understand.

- **This is not a textbook.**
- **This is not a book about menopause.**
- **This is not a book about hysterectomy.**
- **This is not a book on how to grow old gracefully.**
- **This is not a book filled with "a million and one things you can do to have a fulfilling life."**
- **This is not a book to teach you coping skills for those "difficult years."**
- **This book will not tell you to "just get a grip" or tell you "it's all in your head."**
- **This book will not tell you "just eat the right foods and everything will be okay."**

"Well, then, what will this book do?"

This book will acquaint you with an old friend— one present at your conception and with you every step of the way ever since. That friend is your body's natural hormone, estrogen, normally manufactured in your ovaries.

If the quality of your life is important to you, estrogen should remain your best friend for the rest of your life.

What's happening to me?

Chapter 1

Are you wondering what happened to the old you—that reliable, energetic, organized, reasonably content, productive person you used to be? Where did she go?

Lately the woman in your mirror can't remember anything. She's totally disorganized, bogged down, exhausted—a bundle of nerves. Even the simplest conversations have turned into confrontations.

All you know is that your mind just doesn't seem to work anymore. You forget important dates, miss appointments, don't follow through on your commitments. You are tired all the time. You can't seem to remember just what you were supposed to do.

The boss has let you know you'd better shape up—he can't put up with your inefficiency much longer. Your kids are asking each other—and you— "What's wrong ?" How could you begin to explain what is going on? You don't understand it yourself. But you have a terrifying fear that you're losing your mind.

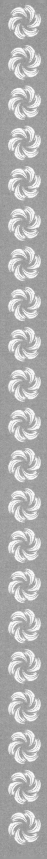

Guess what. The problem probably isn't your mind.

"What is wrong with me?"

One strong possibility exists.

"What's that?"

Something very important. Something that was destined to happen at some time in your life: Pooped-out ovaries.

Your hormone system

In the body of every human being, male and female alike, is an *endocrine system*. This system consists of several glands which produce hormones—special chemicals which help regulate a variety of body functions. These glands include the pituitary glands, the thyroid and parathyroid, the pancreas, adrenal cortex and adrenal medulla, the testes (in men), and (in women) the ovaries. And that's as technical as we are going to get—honest!

Barring any abnormal conditions, these hormone-producing glands keep working throughout our lives. There is, however, one major exception: the ovaries. The ovaries, which began making and circulating a number of hormones at puberty, slow down their function by the time a woman reaches her forties or early fifties. The level of some of those hormones in her body drops to deficiency levels.

14

Let's discuss that process. You need to understand what happens and why, and learn what you can do about it!

Let's start by looking at three important hormones produced in the ovaries: *estrogen, progesterone,*

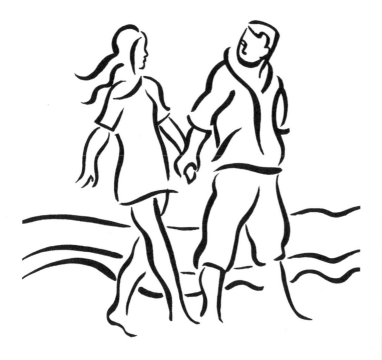

and *testosterone.* These hormones have the most critically important influence on how a woman's body functions. They are manufactured through a complex process involving a number of other hormones, which actually form their "building blocks."

Estrogen and progesterone are called *female hormones,* because they are present in greater quantities in women's bodies than in men's. Similarly, testosterone is called a *male hormone*, because it is present in greater quantities in men's bodies than it is in women's.

Biochemically, all of the ovarian hormones are very closely related to each other, in spite of having different names and playing different roles. They each influence how the other works in the body. Their primary roles are as follows:

Estrogen is the most basic female hormone. Estrogen affects the function of a woman's nervous system, metabolic system, circulatory system, reproductive system, skeletal structure, and skin.

Progesterone is a woman's "control hormone" for menses. It regulates menstruation in the absence of pregnancy.

Testosterone serves the main purpose of regulating a woman's *libido*, or sex drive. There is some evidence that testosterone also helps a woman's sense of well-being.

A deficiency of these three hormones—a lack of them circulating in the blood—causes a variety of problems. Some of these problems are simply annoying. Others are more serious, even life-threatening. This is especially true with estrogen, because that one chemical plays so many roles in keeping a woman's body working properly.

There are a number of natural chemicals in the body that are termed "estrogens," but the active estrogen in the blood as it circulates through the body is known as *estradiol*. This is the form of estrogen the body actually uses, and the form of estrogen we will be discussing throughout the book.

16

Unfortunately, hormone deficiency is programmed into every woman's life.

Ovaries "poop out"—stop producing the necessary amounts of hormones—by the time a woman reaches her forties or early fifties. Some women experience this event earlier than others, and some much later. But the fact remains: it happens to all women, if they live long enough.

Up until this century, estrogen deficiency wasn't much of a problem. That isn't to say that women dealt with the condition better, but that women seldom lived long enough to experience it! It's not a decrease in coping ability, but an increase in life span that makes hormone deficiency, and especially estrogen deficiency, a very real problem for today's woman.

Back in the "good old days," women rarely survived much beyond their fifties. There was no knowledge of what we might consider "mid-life changes" because there were very few occurrences of the condition! But women now are living thirty or forty years after their ovaries stop producing hormones. We have well-documented evidence of what happens when a woman becomes hormone deficient. We know that even though the process is "normal," it leads to pathological—unhealthy—consequences. If left untreated, it causes abnormalities that make the body work less efficiently, with potentially life-threatening consequences.

A is for Attitude.

Chapter 2

Think you need an attitude adjustment? Most of us find it hard to maintain a positive, winning attitude when our bodies are not functioning normally.

Estrogen deficiency promotes the worst in attitudes. Why?

Because estrogen affects a woman's entire body in one way or another. The nervous system, metabolic system, circulatory system, reproductive system, bones and skin are all affected when they don't receive sufficient amounts of estrogen.

The first noticeable signs of estrogen deficiency usually occur in the nervous system and skin, because these two systems depend heavily on estrogen for support and stability. The state of your nervous system determines your ability to cope with everyday stresses and strains. And the condition of your skin affects not only your appearance, but also your comfort... in more ways than one.

For starters, your skin and nervous system combine to form your body's temperature control center. Together, they assess surrounding temperatures and respond accordingly—they make you shiver to gener-

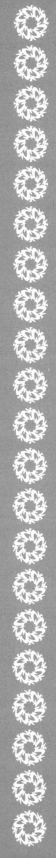

ate heat, or perspire to cool down. A woman experiencing the earliest symptoms of estrogen deficiency is likely to experience inappropriate sensations of heat or cold. She begins having unexpected chills, night sweats, the dreaded hot flashes.

"Won't they ever stop? They wake me up every night, soaking wet from perspiration. My husband and I are always fighting over the air conditioner setting."

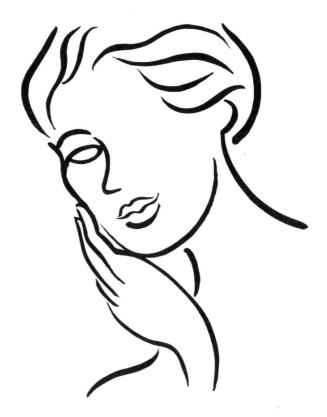

Dry skin—skin lacking its natural lubricants—also becomes a problem. This is more than a cosmetic issue. Dry skin in the vaginal area can make intimacy difficult, if not impossible.

"Every time we have intercourse it's really dry, and it burns and hurts so much we hardly do anything anymore."

So there you have them: the earliest signs of estrogen deficiency:

- **irritability and emotional swings**
- **hot flashes and night sweats**
- **dry skin**
- **pain during intercourse**

Is all that enough to give you a bad attitude or what?

"I get tired just thinking about it. In fact, these days I get tired all the time."

That's not surprising. You probably aren't getting enough sleep!

When you are estrogen deficient, things are going on in your body that can make sleeping difficult. Hot flashes disrupt your normal sleep patterns. If they don't wake you up completely, they bring you up from a deeper, more restful sleep to a lighter, less restful sleep. You may find yourself throwing off the bedcovers, which can disturb your bed partner, who starts tossing and turning and further disturbs your rest.

"We're talking about menopause, aren't we? Isn't menopause inevitable?" Some people say only two things in life are inevitable: death and taxes. Whether these are natural or not, most people benefit from avoiding them as long as possible. And no, we aren't talking about menopause. Menopause is a time period. Estrogen deficiency is the problem. Correcting estrogen deficiency avoids the problems of menopause indefinitely.

21

Another possible sleep disrupter is depression. Estrogen deficient women are often mildly depressed. Depression may cause you to wake up in the middle of the night, make it difficult to fall back into a restful sleep, and/or awaken you earlier in the morning than usual. Even if your sleep patterns are not greatly disturbed, depression itself can make you *feel* chronically fatigued.

Combine a possibly hectic daily routine with loss of sleep and the fatigue of depression and you may have the answer to why you "feel tired all the time." There is no mystery to it at all—it's simply the logical result of the changes going on in your body.

"Well, okay, but a little fatigue won't kill a person. We're talking about a mild depression. How serious can that be?"

Well, that depends on the individual. Fortunately, most women who become estrogen deficient and feel like they're "going crazy" are in no danger of becoming seriously mentally ill. But why suffer any mental or emotional instability? The cure is simply to bring the estrogen in your system back to normal levels.

For most women, it really is just that simple.

B is for Bones.

Chapter 3

Estrogen plays a positive role in the production and protection of bone tissue. Estrogen blocks some of the body's bone-dissolving processes, and stimulates the body's conversion of vitamin D and calcium. When a woman becomes estrogen deficient, her body becomes less efficient at maintaining bone structure. Many of the bone cells that die are not replaced. Her bones become less dense, and thus more weak and brittle. In fact, a woman may lose up to one-half of her bone substance in the first five years of estrogen deficiency. This is the condition known as osteoporosis.

"I've heard of that. Can't you fix osteoporosis by taking calcium or vitamin D supplements?"

No, unfortunately. You cannot prevent or correct bone loss with calcium and vitamin D alone. You must also have enough estrogen in the blood. Estrogen and calcium are like a bricklayer and a pile of bricks. You need both to build a strong wall. So even if bone loss is diagnosed, it cannot be repaired by simply drinking more milk or taking vitamin and mineral supplements. You must also replace the estrogen your body needs.

Calcium and vitamin D are important nutrients.

When you are young, they help you build healthy bones. As you age, however, bone production naturally slows down. Men and women alike achieve peak

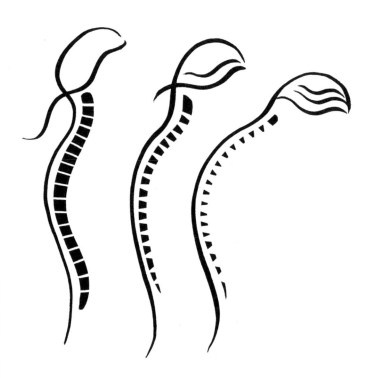

bone mass at about age 35, and gradually lose bone density over the remainder of their lives. Women can lose approximately one-third more bone mass than men, partly because estrogen deficiency affects their bodies' ability to use calcium and vitamin D to maintain their bones.

Bone loss from estrogen deficiency can sneak up on you, because it has no apparent symptoms. A fracture may be the first indication that the bones have become brittle. Brittle, weakened ribs may break during such ordinary activities as coughing or twisting. Minor slips and falls become increasingly dangerous as bones degenerate. Broken arms and wrists happen when people try to "catch" themselves when falling. As people age, they face an increased risk of hip fracture because of their decreased mobility and slower reactions—they are often unable to stop themselves from falling.

Most hip fractures result from falls, but some women have spontaneous hip fractures. They turn quickly, or step off a curb—any motion that places stress on the hip joint. The hip bone is so weak that it snaps, and the woman falls to the ground in terrible pain. The broken bone causes the fall, instead of the fall causing the broken bone. Not a pretty picture, is it? Neither is the sight of a woman crippled by spinal bone collapse.

Spinal bone collapse is one of the most disabling forms of spontaneous bone fracture. The front part of the individual spinal bones (the vertebrae) soften and collapse. As one after another vertebrae flatten, the upper body is forced forward, permanently bent into a position doctors refer to as "dowager's hump." A woman with this problem cannot straighten up because her bones have permanently collapsed. They cannot be repaired. Her back will never again be in its normal position.

Bones weakened and made brittle by estrogen deficiency are dangerous. They are also preventable. Correcting estrogen deficiency protects the body from excessive bone loss.

Some Facts* About Osteoporosis:
(Abnormal thinning of the bones)

1 Osteoporosis causes more than 1,300,000 fractures annually in the United States.

2 The cost of osteoporosis in the United States each year is over 10 billion dollars.

3 Osteoporosis can cause painful spinal fractures, leading to deformity, shrinking of height and disability.

4 Most hip fracture survivors cannot resume their accustomed daily activities without help.

5 One in five victims of hip fractures die within one year of their injury.

6 Four out of five hip fractures occur in women.

*from Consensus Conference in Copenhagen, Denmark, 1990

Dowager's hump is not only awkward and unattractive, but often very painful. For one thing, the bone coverings themselves are very sensitive. The pressure from the fractured bone on the coverings can be very painful. For another, most of the body's major nerve tracts pass through the spinal bones. When these bones collapse, the nerves may become pinched, causing chronic, severe pain that can radiate out into the body parts served by those nerves.

In and of themselves, any of these problems can greatly affect the quality of a woman's life. But it doesn't end there. A major hip fracture may threaten a woman's life. Take a look at the chart on this page. The figures are disturbing, aren't they?

C is for Circulation.

Chapter 4

The human body has a wonderfully efficient system for distributing life-sustaining substances throughout the body: our circulatory system. Nutrients, gases such as oxygen, and natural chemicals of all kinds (hormones, enzymes, electrolytes, sugar and proteins) all circulate in the blood. The blood also picks up waste products from throughout the body, and circulates them to the kidneys, liver and skin for elimination from the body.

One might compare the blood circulation to a water system, with the heart as the central pump. It pushes the blood out to the most distant capillaries and receives the blood back through the veins. It passes through the lungs to take on oxygen and get rid of carbon dioxide (a waste gas).

Endocrine glands in various parts of the body manufacture hormones—including insulin, thyroid, the male and female hormones—and release them directly into the blood as it circulates through those organs.

Every cell in your body is dependent on the routine circulation of your blood. When the flow of blood is blocked, serious problems arise. Blood vessels get clogged or blocked when a substance called *plaque* forms on the inside of them. This substance can slowly collect on the inside of the blood vessels, building up over time, until a blockage forms. It's a lot like grease getting into a sink drain. Over time, that greasy buildup will become so

thick it will slow the drain, or block it completely.

Plaque buildup in the blood vessels can slow the travel of blood, and make your heart work harder to keep circulation going. If the inside of a blood vessel gets too narrow, circulation may stop in that area of the body. If it were to happen in one or more of the *coronary arteries*—the blood vessels in the heart—it could cause a "heart attack." If it were to happen in the brain, it could cause a "stroke."

Clogged blood vessels due to estrogen deficiency can cause life-threatening heart attacks and strokes. They can also be prevented. Correcting estrogen deficiency helps protect you from clogged arteries.

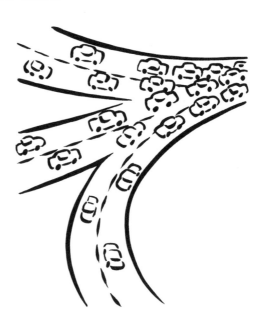

"Why are we talking about all this?"

Because studies have proven that when women become estrogen deficient they are more likely to have clogged blood vessels, heart attacks and strokes. In fact, women who are estrogen deficient have twice as many "heart attacks" as those who are not estrogen deficient. (While this probably is true for "strokes" as well, the final proof is not yet in.)

28

Irregular Periods: Your early warning system.

Chapter 5

Usually, the first indication a woman has that her ovaries are "pooping out" is an irregular menstrual pattern. Progesterone is the hormone that prepares your uterus for pregnancy during the course of the usual ovarian cycle. If pregnancy does not take place, then progesterone helps control the menstrual period. When the ovaries "poop out," ovulation stops. So does any progesterone production. That is why bleeding may become irregular or abnormal at that time.

While this irregular bleeding may be the first sign of impending ovarian failure, your body's estrogen levels may remain at normal levels for quite some time. That explains why you might not yet be experiencing any other signs of hormone deficiency (such as hot flashes, night sweats, or irritability).

If this were the case, you would not yet need estrogen replacement therapy. You would, however, benefit from progesterone replacement. Progesterone would control your irregular periods and help prevent hyperplasia—abnormalities in the lining of the uterus.

Unfortunately, natural progesterone is not widely available for oral use. (A *micronized* form of natural

progesterone is available by special prescription, but it is quite expensive.) A close relative to natural progesterone is used instead: the widely prescribed synthetic medroxyprogesterone acetate (MPA) known by the brand name Provera.

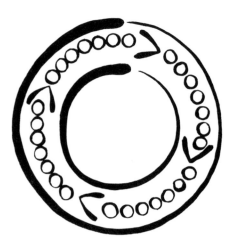

MPA is well-tolerated by most women, although some (fewer than 10%) note PMS-like symptoms. These symptoms are usually related to dosage and may go away when dosage is reduced to the lowest possible level. If not, then MPA should not be used. Other synthetic progesterones are available, including some found in birth control pills—such as norethindrone or norgestrel.

"I've had a hysterectomy. Do I need progesterone?"

No, you do not, according to the latest scientific information. Progesterone is prescribed to protect the lining of the uterus. You do not need progesterone if you do not have a uterus.

Your doctor is the best source of information regarding your need for progesterone.

Estrogen Replacement Therapy.

Chapter 6

If you are having any of the symptoms of estrogen deficiency, discuss them with your doctor. He or she can evaluate your symptoms, perhaps run a few tests, and then make a diagnosis.

Let's assume you and your doctor agree that you are estrogen deficient. What next?

1. **Your doctor needs to write a prescription for estrogen.**

2. **If you still have your uterus, your doctor needs to write another prescription for progesterone. (This will continue buffering the effects of estrogen on the lining of the uterus, as your body has done since puberty.)**

3. **You need to fill both prescriptions and take the hormones.**

It's really that simple… almost.

The first rule of medicine is "do no harm," so before we doctors write any prescriptions, we make sure we're not getting our patients into trouble. Before we prescribe hormone replacement therapy, we go through a safety check process:

31

Are you pregnant?

Don't laugh—it happens!

Are you up to date on your annual exams?
(breast exam, mammogram, pelvic exam, Pap smear and any other tests your doctor feels are needed regularly).

If not, let's do these first.

Have you had any abnormal vaginal bleeding?

If yes, let's do an endometrial sampling to make sure the lining of the uterus is okay. It's a simple office procedure that doesn't take much longer than a Pap smear but may cause some cramping.

Do you have any medical conditions which would prohibit taking these hormones?

These include:

- **recent endometrial cancer (cancer in the lining of the uterus)**

- **breast cancer**

- **acute (active) liver disease**

Do you have a blood clotting disorder?

Your doctor will want to know if you have a rare condition known as acute vascular thrombosis/ embolism—an abnormal clotting condition inside blood vessels. This is a rare medical occurrence usually associated with disease. However, some very rare people seem to be born with a tendency for their normal blood clotting mechanism to go wrong. Its relationship to estrogen is generally associated with high-

32

dose birth control pills and not the estrogen used in estrogen replacement therapy. It is associated with

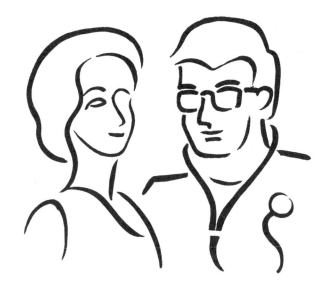

factors which have been shown to be 200-1,000 times stronger when using even today's low-dose birth control pills compared to using natural estrogen. This explains why this condition would not be expected when taking natural estrogen replacement, but why it is an important consideration if a woman has a previous history of this condition.

Once you clear your doctor's "check list," you can safely begin your estrogen replacement therapy.

"How much estrogen will I need?"

Conjugated estrogen 0.625 mg is the minimum needed to protect your **Bones** and help prevent osteoporosis, and to protect your **Circulation** and help prevent heart attacks. (Those were the B and C of our ABC's, remember?) More estrogen may be required to treat the A needs (**Attitude**) for awhile. Women under 45 usually need more estrogen than those over 55, but this depends completely on the individual. A combination of symptoms and blood testing can guide therapy. You and your doctor, working as a team, can determine the best therapy for you.

"What are the prescriptions like?"

Each of the three ovarian hormones come in tablet form to be taken by mouth. Taken properly, these tablets usually successfully replace the hormones your body needs.

"Does that mean these tablets might not work? "

There is something I call the "One-in-Twenty" syndrome. That simply means approximately five percent of the population, or one person in twenty, has a barrier within her body's circulatory system—most likely an extremely good filtration system in her liver— that prevents estrogen taken orally from getting out of her digestive system and into her blood.

This person follows the instructions on her prescription to the letter, but still doesn't feel any better. This stuff was supposed to get rid of those pesky hot flashes and other annoying problems, but doesn't seem to be working!

Back she goes to her doctor, understandably frustrated, saying "These things aren't doing any good." And sure enough, when you check for the active form of estrogen in the blood (serum estradiol)—it is very low, even though she has been taking the tablets faithfully. Since the necessary estrogen is not circulating through the body in the blood, the estrogen deficiency has not been corrected.

"How do you treat women who have this 'One-in-Twenty' syndrome?"

Since oral estrogen enters the blood through the digestive system, women with the "One-in-Twenty" syndrome need to use a different route to replace the estrogen in their blood stream. Higher and higher dosages of oral estrogen will not safely correct their estrogen deficiency.

Too often in years past, a woman who made this complaint would simply be labeled a "complainer." Her very real problems would be dismissed as being "all in her head." After all, the therapy worked just fine for everyone else. Perhaps she should consider some psychiatric therapy.

These doctors weren't mean-spirited—they were uninformed. They had no way of knowing the estrogen they were giving these women was not getting into their blood stream.

We're better educated now. For the past several years we have been able to measure hormone levels in the body by using blood tests. These tests make it possible to measure the active form of estrogen in the blood stream and find out precisely what is happening (or not happening). Those with the "One-in-Twenty" syndrome will have test results showing estrogen deficiency, even though they are swallowing their estrogen

These blood tests were made possible by using some new techniques for which a woman scientist was awarded a Nobel prize a few years ago. It took quite a while for these tests to be available outside research labs. They tend to be rather expensive, and many health care professionals are still unfamiliar with how to use them.

tablets every day just as they were told to do. They (and their doctors) can be assured their problems are in their hormone levels, and not in their heads!

More importantly, since their problems lie in the method of estrogen delivery, they can be solved.

We have come a long way!

There has always been a great deal of confusion in both the general public and the medical community regarding women's hormones, combined with a reluctance to tackle the issue. This situation has been fostered by a number of factors:

1 Until recently, a poor understanding of a woman's need for hormones and their value in her daily life

2 Until recently, a lack of scientific knowledge to prove that value

3 Until recently, poor testing methods for diagnosis and treatment of estrogen deficiency

4 An emphasis on curing disease rather than *dis-ease*

5 A health care system which rewards health care professionals for *fighting* disease rather than *preventing* disease

6 For health care professionals, the time-consuming and frustrating nature of "hormone problems"

7 Generations of folklore about the menopause being something you just have to "get through" (a medieval badge of courage, so to speak — as if PMS, menstruation and childbirth weren't enough!)

Alternative routes to the same end.

Chapter 7

Should oral estrogen replacement therapy prove ineffective, several alternative routes are currently available. Each has points to recommend it, as well as one or two less favorable characteristics:

Skin Patches: Skin patches permit the estrogen to be absorbed through the skin. They are very simple to use. The estrogen patches are small (about the size of a fifty-cent piece) and as thin as a piece of paper, with adhesive on one side. They are usually placed on the back or lower abdomen, and changed every 3½ days.

When transdermal skin patches were first announced, many of us thought they would be the ideal method for estrogen replacement therapy. However, many women experience problems with the patches. Some women develop an irritating skin rash from the patch. Others find that the patches fall off when they shower or bathe, or when they perspire.

Shots: Shots (intramuscular injections) can be very effective, but are not widely used for a variety of reasons. First, most people don't enjoy receiving injections. Second, they require frequent visits to the doc-

tor's office, as they must be administered every three or four weeks. Third, this method of delivery calls for frequent testing, to determine the amount of estrogen circulating in the body.

With shots, estrogen levels vary widely during the three or so weeks of each dosage. Blood levels of estrogen are highest immediately after each injection

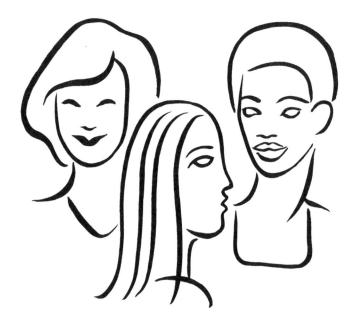

and gradually decrease over the following weeks. Since different women use up the estrogen from the shots at different rates, levels need to be closely watched at first to assure the correct dosage.

Women may hear from older women that the shots "weren't reliable." Although that's no longer the case, it once was true. Reliable testing procedures to help regulate the proper estrogen level have only become available within the past ten years or so.

Vaginal Creams: Vaginal creams have been available for many years. The estrogen is in a cream base, which is placed high in the vagina by means of an applicator. This method is used at night, so that the estrogen can be absorbed through the walls of the vagina and into the blood.

The amount of estrogen absorbed into the blood depends upon the type of estrogen in the cream. For example, *estradiol* may be more effectively absorbed through the vaginal wall than *conjugated estrogen*. Both forms of estrogen have a good local effect on the wall of the vagina. (That means they help soften and lubricate the skin there.)

This method only has two drawbacks. First, the creams can be messy, and may make it necessary to wear panty liners. Second, some women feel uncomfortable about inserting the cream into the vagina.

Vaginal Tablets: It may surprise you to know that vaginal tablets ("pills") are not generally available as such. However, it has been shown that pure estradiol-type estrogen tablets, meant for oral use, can also correct estrogen deficiency when used vaginally. Women using this method must be willing to place a small tablet high in the vagina about three times per week. This placement may be a barrier to some who find it difficult to reach or who have some other objection to putting things into their vagina.

Experience has shown this to be a very useful option, however. For many women, the vaginal tablets are so well absorbed that their dosage can be reduced. For instance, one tablet three times a week vaginally may provide the same results as the identical tablet taken every day by mouth.

Vaginal Rings: Similar to a contraceptive diaphragm, the estradiol vaginal rings are used for three months each. This method is not available in the United States.

Skin Gels: Skin gels are applied to the skin of the upper body on a daily basis. While available in Europe, this method is not available in the United States.

Estrogen Pellets: Small pellets placed under the skin will offer a very promising delivery form for estrogen in the future. These implants are being used successfully in other countries, and are currently undergoing clinical testing in the United States. They will not be available for doctors in the United States to prescribe, however, until they complete the lengthy federal approval process.

This method releases controlled amounts of estrogen slowly and evenly over a period of several months. It does require a simple office procedure to place—and periodically replace—the implant under the skin. It offers long-term convenience, but you cannot change the dosage without removing the implant and replacing it with another.

One way or another, your estrogen deficiency can be treated successfully. All that is needed is good, honest communication between you and your doctor.

So... I have to take medicine?

Chapter 8

When your body manufactures hormones in its endocrine system, and then dumps them into your blood, do you consider those chemicals to be "medicine"? Maybe you should. It might help you appreciate what a great manufacturing marvel the human body is! After all, medicine can be defined as a "healing substance," and your body manufactures a variety of those every minute of the day.

Estrogen is only one of several hormones manufactured by your endocrine system. These hormones, working along with your nervous system, control the activities of every organ and tissue in your body. Without these special chemicals, you could not live.

- **Hormones enable your lungs to extract oxygen from the air and transfer it to your blood stream.**
- **Hormones enable your digestive organs to extract nutrients from the foods you eat and convert them to your body's energy source.**

- **Hormones enable your nervous system to regulate every body movement, and enable your brain to store and process information.**

- **Hormones enable your skeleton to form and support your every movement.**

- **Hormones enable your muscles to grow and move.**

Hormones are essential to your life. Every vital function in your body is dependent on the presence of these chemicals—"medicines," if you will—manufactured in your body.

Sometimes our body does not produce the correct amount of a certain hormone, such as insulin. When that happens, our body cannot work efficiently. We go to our doctors for treatment, and are given medication to correct the problem. We begin taking insulin to replace the amount our body is no longer producing. While we may wish our body was doing the job all by itself, we appreciate having an alternative, because we know we must have the hormone in our body to continue living.

"But estrogen seems… different. I'm just not comfortable talking about it."

People don't have trouble discussing thyroid, or insulin, or other body hormones, but mention estrogen and the conversation screeches to an abrupt halt. Why? Because people know it's a female hormone, and think it has something to do with

42

menopause... and both those things are related to sex—a subject our parents taught us to avoid.

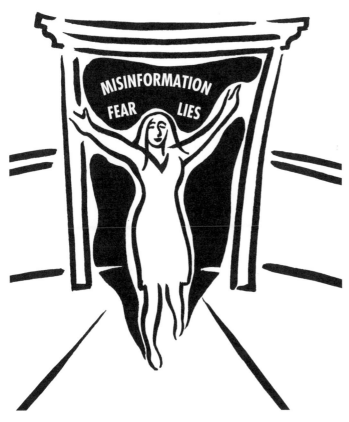

Because people once associated it with "female problems," estrogen deficiency was never discussed in polite society.

In the past, people simply didn't feel comfortable discussing anything that had to do with sex. The subject was spoken of only in hurried, whispered conversations. Women ignorant of scientific facts shared folklore, old wives tales and home

43

remedies. Mostly, they shared in the consequences of their mutual ignorance: the dreaded event known as "menopause."

Fortunately, hormones are no longer a forbidden subject, even though mentioning them might have made your great-grandparents blush. Estrogen is one of your most essential hormones. As we have already seen, its presence in your body is vitally important to your nerve function, skeletal strength, and blood circulation.

Estrogen deficiency is treatable. The results of estrogen deficiency—all those wretched symptoms we associate with menopause—are preventable. All that is needed is estrogen replacement therapy.

All you need to do is continue receiving the same hormone you've been receiving since puberty. All that you would be changing with estrogen replacement therapy would be the manufacturing source and delivery method.

If that makes replacement estrogen a medicine, well then, so be it! The end result is the same: your blood stream once again carries this life-sustaining chemical to the parts of your body that depend upon it for continued health!

How much is enough?

Chapter 9

How do you determine the level of estrogen needed to prevent estrogen deficiency? Most women—and their health care professionals—have no idea. But that doesn't mean that the answer is unknown, just that most people are unaware of it.

"Can you explain it to me?"

Sure. Let's start with the terminology. Blood levels of estrogen are measured in picograms per milliliter, usually abbreviated to pg/mL.

Now, milliliters are pretty small. They weigh only one gram each, and it takes 5 of them to fill a teaspoon. If you've done any cooking, you can picture about how much volume a milliliter has.

A picogram is infinitely smaller, however. It weighs only one trillionth of a gram, and you could only see it through a high-powered microscope.

When we measure the estrogen level in the blood, we call it the serum estradiol level. So if we put all of these terms together to say a woman's "serum estradiol level is 100," that means there are 100 picograms (trillionths of a gram) of estrogen per milliliter (one-fifth teaspoonful) of her blood.

"Okay. Then what should a woman's serum estradiol level be?"

Throughout a woman's menstruating years (except during pregnancy) her estrogen level usually varies

45

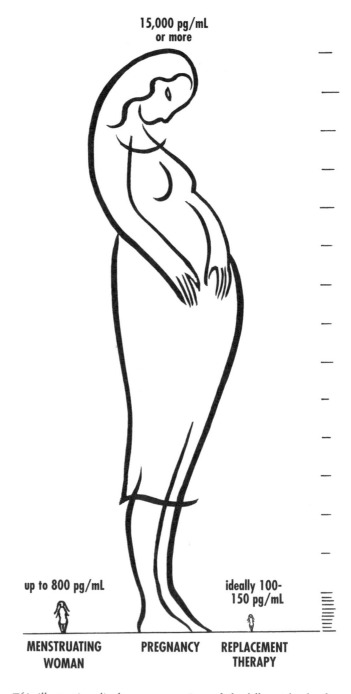

15,000 pg/mL
or more

up to 800 pg/mL

ideally 100-
150 pg/mL

MENSTRUATING WOMAN

PREGNANCY

REPLACEMENT THERAPY

This illustration displays a comparison of the different levels of estradiol in a woman's blood stream at various stages in her life.

from about 40 pg/mL to about 800 pg/mL, depending on the time in her monthly cycle. Levels are at their lowest just before and just after the start of the menstrual period each month. Levels are at their highest about a week earlier in her cycle.

Estrogen deficiency is said to occur when a woman's serum estradiol level drops and remains below 60. This is the minimum level women need for a beneficial effect on bones and circulation. (It also seems reasonable to say that estrogen deficiency would become severe should the level drop below normal levels for men, which many laboratories report as being up to 70 picograms per milliliter.)

"How much estrogen does a woman actually need?"

A good rule of thumb is to maintain the estradiol level between 60 and 150, while understanding that some people may need a higher level for a while.

Studies show the minimum level needed to prevent osteoporosis appears to be 60-70. A level above 100 appears to protect the blood vessels, as well. Higher levels may be necessary to eliminate such symptoms as hot flashes, night sweats, insomnia, or irritability. This is especially true in younger women (those under the age of 50, although this designation is arbitrary).

More is not necessarily "better." The goal is simply to restore your body's estrogen level to that necessary to maintain normal body function. There is no need to waste money by taking more estrogen than necessary. (But don't slight yourself by taking less than you need.)

"How do you know the dosage is correct?"

After you have been on estrogen replacement thera-

47

Other tests are sometimes appropriate, as well. Certain X-ray procedures can help your doctor analyze your bone density. A special urine test can provide information on bone regeneration. And another type of blood test can show your cholesterol levels. Your doctor will advise you about these tests.

py for a few weeks, your doctor will meet with you to discuss how the therapy is working. If you had been having problems with hot flashes, night sweats or irritability, you will probably have a good idea as to whether or not the therapy is helping those symptoms.

Special laboratory tests that measure the serum estradiol level in your blood stream are necessary to determine precisely what is taking place within your body, however.

"So, will I start feeling better right away?"

Timing of the tests is important. Hormone levels in your body vary from week to week, or even throughout different hours of the day, depending on the type of hormone replacement therapy you are receiving. To obtain the most accurate results, your doctor will probably ask you to schedule your blood tests according to certain "rules of thumb," as outlined in the table on the following page.

Once your serum estradiol levels are returned to normal, you should feel better. Any symptoms of estrogen deficiency (night sweats, hot flashes, etc.) you have been experiencing should taper off. And you should notice your mental and emotional outlook returning to normal as well.

If you are feeling worse rather than better when taking hormone replacement therapy, talk to your doctor. Something needs correcting.

"What are the chances of this happening?"

Very, very slight. But any form of medication, like all other substances in life (foods, chemicals, pollens), can trigger a rare reaction due to an allergy or individual sensitivity. The most common instances of sensitivity to estrogen replacement compounds we have seen over the years have been related to ingredients other than the estrogen itself.

Some people are sensitive to dyes—yellow dye, especially. Some are sensitive to the "binder" in a tablet (the substance that holds the powdered ingredients together in tablet form). Some are sensitive to the type of oil base used in an injectable form.

Such sensitivities are very rare, and like all allergic

If the type of therapy you are receiving is:

Tablets

> Have the blood test either several hours after the last dose, or just before the next dose is due. (For the results to be accurate, you need to have been on the same dosage level for at least two weeks.)

Patches

> Have the blood test on the 2nd or 3rd day of a patch (they are changed every 3½ days).

Shots

> Since the shot lasts about 3 weeks, it helps to get a 'halfway level' 10 days after the shot. (The estrogen in your blood is highest right after the shot and then gradually drops off.)

Vaginal Cream

> Test 12-24 hours after application.

---

reactions, often hard to recognize. The symptoms may be bizarre, and very disturbing to the individual having them. They may include headaches, tiredness, itching, skin rash, difficulty concentrating, or trouble sleeping.

Once identified, allergy or sensitivity symptoms can be quickly corrected. Such symptoms will improve (or disappear) once you stop taking the offending substance and switch to another form of medication—one which does not include the ingredient to which you are allergic. Say, for instance, you have an allergy to yellow dye. Switching from a yellow tablet to a white tablet of the same medication should make your symptoms disappear.

If you begin experiencing strange symptoms after starting hormone replacement therapy, call your doctor's office and insist on making an appointment for a discussion. Make sure your doctor understands what you are saying.

Insist on a reasonable explanation for the symptoms you are experiencing. Or request a change in therapy to a form of hormone to which you are not sensitive. There are many options available.

Why is this so important? Because hormone replacement therapy will enhance the quality of your life. It will help protect your bones and your circulation for the rest of your life. And it will improve the way you feel about your life. Discontinuing hormone replacement therapy because of a rare but "fixable" sensitivity to a particular compound of the medication might alleviate your allergy symptoms, but would definitely leave your attitude, bones and circulation in jeopardy.

Talk to your doctor if you experience problems with any aspect of your hormone replacement therapy. You and your doctor, working as a team, can find the source of the problem. Together, you can make the therapy work for you, the way it is intended to.

Do I have to have periods?

Chapter 10

Cyclic menstrual bleeding usually stops some-time between the ages of 45 and 55. Most women don't miss this monthly ritual. After all, menstruation serves only one physiologic function: it prepares the body for pregnancy.

More specifically, the ovarian hormones stimu-late the endometrium (the lining of the uterus), preparing it to receive a fertilized egg. If an egg is fer-tilized during this cycle, the woman may become pregnant, the endometrium serving as a "nest" for the developing embryo over the nine months of preg-nancy. If no egg is fertilized, the lining is sloughed off, and the woman menstruates.

It's a somewhat messy process, but highly efficient and extremely important. Becoming a woman depends both symbolically and physiologically on this exact cyclic hormone function. Yet once the menstrual peri-ods stop, it is certainly understandable that a person doesn't want to start the mess up again voluntarily.

We know that a major reason women rebel against hormone replacement therapy is the chance of contin-

51

ued period-like bleeding. And in fact, one aspect of hormone therapy may temporarily restore cyclic bleed-

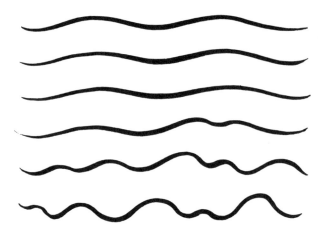

ing. When progesterone is taken in cycles (10-12 days out of the month), then period-like bleeding usually will occur. This bleeding may decrease as time passes, or may continue indefinitely.

The good news is that there is an alternative strategy which may stop the bleeding. We have found that having women take their estrogen and progesterone together, in 25 days-per-month cycles, brings most bleeding to a stop within a few months. We know that this is a safe and effective alternative to the cycling that causes monthly periods.

"What about pregnancy?"

Hormone replacement therapy is not a birth control method. It will neither make you fertile nor prevent conception. Unless you have had a tubal ligation or hysterectomy, or your partner has had a vasectomy, you need to discuss this important subject with your doctor.

"What about PMS?"

We mentioned that some women taking MPA progesterone might have some PMS-like symptoms. If that becomes a problem, there are several strategies to try:

- **Decrease the dose as much as possible.**
- **Change from 10-12 day cycles of MPA progesterone to every day, but at the lowest dose possible.**
- **Change to a different type of synthetic progesterone or consider the *micronized* form (even though it is hard to find and rather expensive).**
- **Consider not taking progesterone after all.**

That last one may sound obvious, but remember: progesterone protects your uterine lining. *Not taking progesterone puts a woman more at risk of endometrial cancer.* Although the increased risk is small, far less than the risk of heart attacks, strokes, broken bones, etc., that would arise if a woman discontinued taking her estrogen replacement therapy because of intolerance to the progesterone she was taking along with it, it cannot be ignored.

While your doctor has methods to detect and treat early warning signs of overgrowth (hyperplasia) or cancer in the lining of the uterus, a satisfactory way of taking progesterone can almost always be found. Your doctor is your best source of information and advice on the subject of progesterone.

Close contact with your doctor may be required to reassure you and answer any questions or concerns you may have when you first start taking hormones.

53

Please don't take my ovaries!

Chapter 11

Let's talk for a minute about a special situation which brings on a sudden ovarian failure and instant estrogen deficiency: the removal of a woman's ovaries at the time of a hysterectomy.

It is important to understand the consequences of the decision to take out or leave the ovaries at the time of hysterectomy. Let's think about this situation for a minute. What really happens when the ovaries are both removed?

Well, no one will argue that nothing happens. It's true that one unique function is lost forever: the ability to procreate. However, procreation depends upon an intact uterus. We're discussing removing the ovaries along with the uterus. Unless one wished to donate an egg for surrogate parenting, procreation would not be possible anyway.

Removal of the ovaries also means a wonderful hormone manufacturing source is lost. Once a woman's ovaries are removed, her primary hormone manufacturing plant is shut down and she

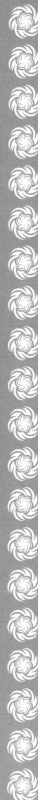

55

must rely on estrogen replacement from that point on.

However, ovarian removal (oophorectomy) is sometimes the best way to manage a woman's health. Two scenarios are very common:

What if the ovaries were already damaged by disease or malfunction? A woman's doctor might

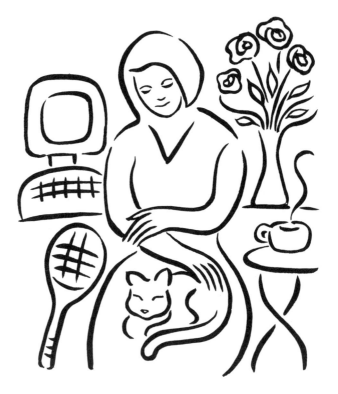

advise that such ovaries be removed at the time of her hysterectomy.

And what about a woman facing a hysterectomy after her procreating and hormone manufacturing processes have stopped—after her ovaries have already begun to "poop out"? When a woman is nearing that time in her life, her doctor may also recommend removing her ovaries at the time of her hysterectomy.

Open communication with your doctor is always important. If your doctor recommends removal of your uterus, you should know the reasons behind that recommendation and understand them fully before agreeing to the surgery. Likewise, if your doctor recommends removal of your ovaries during that same surgery, you should have a good understanding of the reasons for that recommendation.

These facts should reassure you:

- **We do not recommend removal of your ovaries without good medical reason.**

- **We do not remove your ovaries without your permission.**

- **Neither natural ovarian failure nor surgical removal of the ovaries should change you—your essential nature—in any way, if your estrogen is restored to normal levels with estrogen replacement therapy.**

Some straight talk about sex.

Chapter 12

Sex is difficult to discuss, isn't it? Many people have questions that go unanswered, even in the privacy of their doctor's office. The reasons for their bashfulness could fill another entire book. All I want to do here in this brief chapter is present a few hormonal "facts of life."

Fact #1: In order for there to be normal sexual activity, two conditions must exist:

- **An individual must have normal sexual apparatus. (In "mechanical" terms, the parts must be in good repair and well lubricated.)**
- **Second, that individual must have a desire for sexual activity.**

Fact #2: There must be no psychiatric, psychological, or physical barriers present to prevent normal sexual activity.

Now, isn't that simple?

Notice we haven't defined "normal" or told you who your partner should be. That's your business. We have simply said that if an individual is free of inhibi-

59

tions and illness (whether mental or physical), only two conditions must be met.

"What does this have to do with a discussion of hormones?"

Well, we need to discuss another of the hormones produced by your ovaries: the male hormone, testosterone. Testosterone has a definite influence on your libido (your desire for sexual activity). You do not need testosterone to function sexually or to be satisfied by sexual activity, but it does influence your *desire* for sex.

If your testosterone level is low, you may simply lose your normal interest in sexual activity.

Keep in mind that we are talking about an otherwise normal environment. If your partner smells bad, or is abusive; if you are depressed or stressed out; if there is no privacy... then who needs it, right? Raising your testosterone level will not overcome such understandable barriers to sexual desire.

However, women who have always had a normal libido but then seem to have lost it could ask their doctors to check their testosterone level.

"Why haven't I ever heard of this before?"

This is relatively new information! Research typically follows money, and there has been no profit motivation in studying the female libido. (While there have been isolated studies since the 40's and 50's, only recently has research started to catch up with this problem.) Combine that factor with the common acceptance of all the myths associated with aging and it is possible to build a wall of professional indifference.

A few years ago we ran two computerized searches of recent worldwide medical literature on this subject. We found fewer than a half-dozen articles—and those

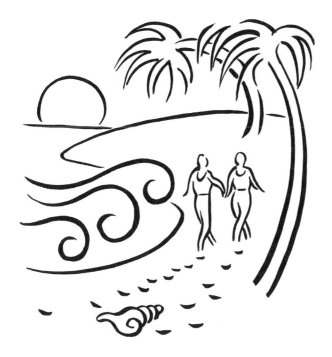

were found in the oncology (study of cancer) and psychiatric fields. What prompted our search was a drastic loss of libido we had frequently observed in young women following the removal of their ovaries due to pelvic disease.

Now, doctors have been trained for generations to believe that any male hormone should keep a woman's

Your sex life need not "poop out" when your ovaries do. Testosterone replacement therapy can help you maintain your normal desire for sex.

libido normal. Since other sites in the body manufacture male hormones, it was thought that losing the ovaries was not important to sexual functioning.

WRONG!

Testosterone is apparently the only male hormone that influences libido in women, and the ovaries are a major source for testosterone production in women. So when the ovaries are removed or fail to produce enough testosterone—GUESS WHAT? Bye-bye, libido!

"How can I find out if I have a testosterone deficiency?"

A blood test for testosterone is available. This test can be done in any full-service medical laboratory and should be relatively inexpensive.

Normal levels may vary slightly from lab to lab; but in menstrual age women the approximate range is 20-90 ng/100mL. (That's 20-90 nanograms per 100 milliliters of blood. A nanogram is one billionth of a gram, and a milliliter is one-fifth of a teaspoonful.)

There are major differences between men's and women's levels. Comparably aged men have a range of 300-1200. In other words, the highest normal level for women is less than one-third the lowest normal level for men. This disparity is not surprising. Testosterone acts in men as their dominant gonadal hormone. Only a small amount in women "fine tunes" their system.

"What can be done about testosterone deficiency?"

There are commercial combination tablets available, combining estrogen and testosterone. But some have found these tablets to be unreasonably expensive or providing inappropriate dosages for women. We have had good success using generic methyl testosterone. Methyl testosterone, available in a 10 mg. tablet, can often be given two or three days a week with good response. Your doctor will need to prescribe for you. The number of days per week can be decreased or increased, according to the results obtained. It's advisable to stay with any dose at least two weeks before changing. (We have never had to give more than one tablet per day, nor less than one tablet per week.) Most people get along well with the two or three days per week schedule.

"Will taking testosterone give me masculine characteristics?"

If the testosterone level is maintained in the normal range for women, there is no reason to believe that a woman's voice would deepen or she would sprout whiskers or any other such problem.

If a woman suspects testosterone replacement is causing some problems, she should contact her doctor and discuss the situation. As with estrogen replacement, blood testing can always be done to guide testosterone replacement therapy. (Our experience has shown good results by keeping the testosterone level between 50-70 ng/100mL.) If problems persist, the medication could be stopped to see if the symptoms disappear.

63

What about cancer?

Chapter 13

Only one cancer has been shown to have a significant relationship to ovarian hormones. It starts in the lining of the uterus and is known as endometrial cancer. The chance of getting endometrial cancer can be decreased below the expected rate by modern hormone replacement therapy.

Several facts about this disease need to be emphasized:

- **Endometrial cancer is relatively rare (one case per 5,000 in women of all ages; one case per 1,000 in women over 50).**

- **Women who have had a hysterectomy are in no danger of endometrial cancer, since the uterus and its lining are no longer present.**

- **Ideal hormone replacement therapy in women who still have their uterus includes both female hormones (estrogen and progesterone). Including progesterone counteracts the stimulating effect of estrogen on the uterine lining, and reduces the rate of cancer in the uterine lining.**

- **If indicated, a simple office procedure can be used to monitor the condition of the uterine lining. This**

65

procedure can be done at the time of a woman's annual Pap smear appointment and can detect early warning signs before cancer starts.

- **The rare occurrences of endometrial cancer during hormone replacement therapy are usually of a less aggressive form. Because the woman is taking hormone replacement under medical supervision, such cancers are discovered earlier and are almost always cured by hysterectomy.**

Once again, it is very important to have a comfortable working relationship with your doctor. Adding progesterone to your treatment program is a good way to prevent endometrial cancer, but there is the issue of bleeding.

As we mentioned previously, some women resume period-like bleeding if progesterone is added in higher doses for a shorter time (MPA 5-10 mg. daily for 10-12 days each month). If the dose is lowered (MPA 2.5 mg.) and given continuously, then eventually the bleeding will stop for most of these women—but may start up again in the second year of use.

The good news is, most of these women will respond to a 25 day-per-month treatment program of otherwise continuous estrogen and progesterone.

You can see how important it is to have a physician who is interested and knowledgeable and willing to work with you to tailor the best program for your needs. Hormone replacement therapy can get somewhat complex for some women. Working together with your doctor can work for you.

"What about breast cancer?"

For many years, uncertainty and controversy swirled around the possible relationship between

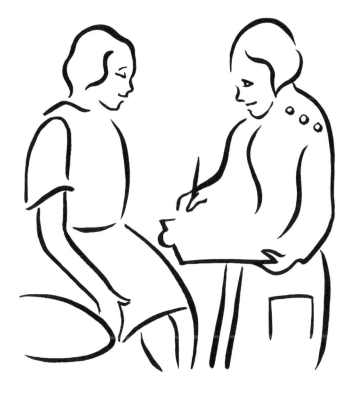

estrogen replacement therapy and breast cancer. Women's magazines, newspapers and television news hosted an information circus, pandering to our deepest fears. Why? Because a number of studies by a variety of experts all seemed to generate conflicting data.

However, we now have huge volumes of evidence, and the news is more and more reassuring.

It is true that some investigators have felt estrogen may increase the risk of breast cancer, especially in women with a family history of breast cancer or in women who have taken estrogen over a long period of time. It is important to understand that the statistics these investigators are weighing represent the difference between a very small risk and no risk at all. In other words, none of these scientists feels that there is anything but a possible, small increase in risk, if any.

Recent evidence is increasingly reassuring. It seems to point squarely at no increased risk at all for the type of hormone replacement therapy currently used in the United States—even for those with a family history of breast cancer.

Three additional notes are worth consideration:

- **The longest reported study to date in which selected women either took hormones or did not provided very interesting results. After 22 years of study, the women taking hormones had no occurrence of breast cancer. Those women not taking hormones had an 11% breast cancer rate—the identical** expected percentage in the general population.

- Although there continues to be a belief that estrogen should not be given to women who have had breast cancer, there is no foundation of proof for that idea. This is an idea which seemed logical in its inception and has been perpetuated through tradition, but which has no evidence whatsoever behind it! In fact, some very prestigious experts have presented forceful arguments in very highly regarded medical journals calling for a re-thinking of this notion. The most important aspect of this debate: the fact that heart and blood vessel disease (which might be prevented by estrogen replacement) presents a much greater risk than any influence of estrogen on the breast, even in women with previously treated breast cancers.

- There is convincing evidence that women who were taking replacement estrogen when they were diagnosed with breast cancer actually have a lower mortality rate than those who were not taking estrogen replacement.

Each woman must decide for herself about this important issue, but current evidence shows no increased risk of breast cancer in estrogen users—and a definite decreased risk from other serious diseases.

Avoiding hormone replacement therapy because of a fear of cancer actually places a woman's life in greater danger—from heart attacks, strokes and serious bone fractures. All of those risk factors can be drastically cut by hormone replacement therapy.

What about those package inserts?

Chapter 14

Have you ever read a pharmaceutical package insert? Package inserts are sheets of information required by the U.S. Food & Drug Administration (FDA). They are placed in the container of medication by the manufacturer and are intended as quick references for health professionals who prescribe or dispense these medications. A large book published annually contains copies of the package inserts for every medication currently available. This book is the *Physician's Desk Reference*, commonly referred to as the "P.D.R."

Some states (California, for example) have regulations unique to estrogen-containing medications, requiring this insert be given directly to the consumer. No other medications have such a requirement. Some people feel this is a political move which misinforms lay people who are not in a position to properly interpret the information or place it in proper perspective.

These regulations are the result of political pressure for protection of women. We have seen

how the early days of estrogen treatment certainly had their problems. There were occasional side effects from the high dosages of **synthetic** estrogen formulated in the early birth control pills; there were occasional side effects from natural estrogen when not buffered with progesterone. The media ran with every scare story, and people began losing confidence in the health care community.

Research intensified and answers emerged. But the public remained skeptical. They didn't know whom to trust. There was increasing pressure on Congress and the FDA to take steps to protect women from possible bad outcomes from estrogen prescriptions. The politicians and bureaucrats responded by requiring an information sheet—a package insert—be included in each and every prescription of any estrogen-containing product.

Now, these information sheets are nothing new. Every single drug sold in America—whether prescription or over-the-counter— has one. And they all look intimidating! They explain the chemical composition of the compound. They explain what the drug does—how it is designed to act on specific parts of the body. They explain what the drug doesn't do—how it doesn't cause baldness or reduce sperm counts, or whatever other tests the drug has had to pass before being allowed to be sold. The sheets then provide documentation of clinical trials, showing how many people took how much of the compound with what measurable results. They explain when the drug is recommended, for what specific purposes, and in what dosages. They explain what to do in case of an overdose. They tell you what sizes or quantities the drug comes in, and the best temperatures at which to store. They even tell you the letters printed or embossed on a tablet. It is a lot of information, all in very fine print. All of the information is useful to pharmacists and physicians, and of possible interest to people taking the drug, depending on how involved they choose to be in their own health care.

But then these inserts get a little scary. They list every negative reaction remotely possible from administration of the drug—no matter how rare. These may be minor, such as headaches or brittle fingernails. Some may be more serious—perhaps dizziness, or an increased heart rate. Some might even be potentially life threatening.

Most disturbing: sometimes the information provided is out of date. In the case of estrogen, some of the listed problems have since been proven not to be caused by natural estrogen at all!

Still, every pharmaceutical manufactured carries such a product information sheet—even acetaminophen. If you read all the rare and obscure things associated with that, you might never treat another headache! But only estrogen prescriptions are required by law to provide that information sheet directly to the consumer. Everything else remains on file at the pharmacy. This is not a conspiracy to keep patients ignorant, but a carefully considered approach to protecting patients from reacting out of ignorance!

"But isn't this kind of information important?"

It is important that physicians understand all of the possible outcomes from any treatment they recommend to their patients. They are trained to analyze the information and keep it in its proper perspective. One negative outcome per 1,000,000 patients is statistically meaningful only to that one individual. You have to balance that against 999,999 other lives significantly enhanced or possibly even saved by that same treatment.

But that's not how most of us are conditioned to view things. We see "possible adverse reactions" and we assume the worst. We begin to fear our health care professionals are out to kill us instead of cure us. It's not rational, but it is human nature.

Suppose every car dealer had to post a window sticker listing everything that had ever happened to anyone while riding in a car. How safe would you feel driving one of those cars off the lot?

"Why do the drug companies go along with this? Aren't they afraid women will refuse to buy their product?"

In one way, the manufacturers benefit from enclosing the information sheet in the estrogen package. Doing so protects them as much as it protects the consumer. They can say, "If you're willing to follow your doctor's advice and take this stuff now that you've read all this, don't blame us if anything goes wrong. We tried to warn you!"

With millions of women taking hormone products there are ample opportunities for something

If you really want to see the information on the package inserts for any drug you have ever taken, visit your public library and ask to see the Physician's Desk Reference. All of these sheets are reproduced in this massive book, and updated every year.

to happen that someone might consider an "adverse reaction." A huge lawsuit could quickly follow. Whether or not there was any merit to the suit would not reduce the enormous cost of defending it in court. Anything which helps place blame elsewhere would be a useful tool.

"Why do so many women question the safety of estrogen?"

Most questions about estrogen safety arise out of problems associated with birth control pills. Birth control pills contain **synthetic** (**un**natural) estrogen and **synthetic** (**un**natural) progesterones. There is a vast difference between the **natural** estrogen prescribed in estrogen replacement therapy and the synthetic estrogen prescribed in birth control pills.

Synthetic estrogen is just what it sounds like: an artificial chemical compound. Natural estrogen is derived from a natural source, and is identical to the estrogen made in a woman's own body. It is the same type of estrogen your body has been exposed to all your life, starting with extremely high doses while you were still in your mother's womb. (Remember our saying normal estradiol levels reach as high as 800 during a woman's natural monthly cycle? During pregnancy a woman's levels reach 15-30 thousand.)

The potency of synthetic estrogen in birth control pills is very high compared to the potency of natural estrogen normally prescribed for estrogen replacement therapy. Even today's "low dose" birth control pills contain **six times** the estrogen potency of the usually advised 0.625 mg of conjugated (natural) estrogen.

The amount of synthetic estrogen in the "low dose" birth control pills has at least two hundred times the influence on liver proteins that natural estrogens have. These liver proteins are probably responsible for the unusually high blood pressure and blood clotting problems (thrombophlebitis) that occur in rare individuals taking birth control pills. These people were probably born with a unique sensitivity to these substances, which manifests itself when they take birth control pills.

If we consider these birth control pills safe, consider how much safer the much lower dosage of natural estrogen in estrogen replacement therapy must be.

Still, to be extra-safe, we advise women who have a history of thrombophlebitis to avoid the oral form of natural estrogen replacement and use a patch or other non-oral delivery method. Non-oral forms of estrogen delivery have the least effect on the liver's production of blood clotting agents.

Estrogen increases your safety.

Chapter 15

Safety can be defined as "freedom from danger, risk and injury," or as "reducing danger or harm." If you think about it, the former is impossible. There simply is no such thing as absolute freedom from risk. You can most certainly lower your risks, and reduce danger or harm, however. Correcting estrogen deficiency by taking natural estrogen replacement does just that. It reduces danger and harm. It's that simple.

When you become estrogen deficient, your greatest danger stems from cardiovascular problems. You face an increased risk of heart attack. What cuts your risk of having a heart attack in half? Natural estrogen replacement!

Your next greatest danger comes from the weakening of your bones. What greatly reduces bone loss, spinal collapse and bone fractures—and thus prevents painful disability and possible death? Natural estrogen replacement!

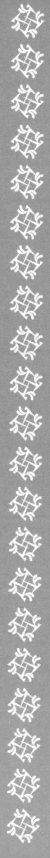

How about hot flashes, night sweats, insomnia, chronic irritability, etc., due to estrogen deficiency? Is there any harm in them? You bet there is! Harm to the quality of your life, and the lives of everyone close to you. These symptoms cause both mental and physical pain.

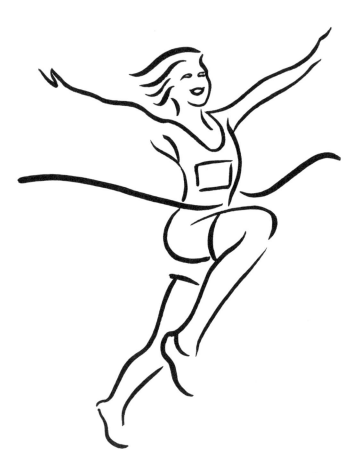

The only person truly able to feel pain is the person suffering it. It's impossible for anyone else to feel it. This explains why we feel so alone when we are in pain. And this is what makes women so vulnerable to those who dismiss their suffering, or deny the severity of what they are experiencing. It's easy for someone not experiencing pain to minimize it.

The dangers of estrogen deficiency are real. The symptoms you feel from estrogen deficiency are real. The myth of menopause as a "change of life" you need to buck up and get through somehow is unreal. And the fear of taking "medication" that could ease your suffering because it might carry "risks" is unreal.

More than twenty years of research and documentation attest to the reality of estrogen deficiency and its profound effect upon a woman's body. The profound restorative effect of natural estrogen replacement therapy has been researched and documented over those years. Why are we still so misinformed on these subjects?

Because fear and suspicion (backed by centuries of myth and misinformation) sell more magazines than facts and reassurance, we have been inundated with sensational headlines and garbled articles on rare occurrences that are made to sound commonplace.

Are there risks or dangers in driving or riding in a car, bus, train or plane? Of course.

Where is the real risk for those with estrogen deficiency? The real risk when you are estrogen deficient lies in not correcting that deficiency.

Are there risks or dangers in shopping at the mall, going to the grocery store, or stopping at a convenience store? Of course.

Are there risks or dangers in staying home? Naturally. A high percentage of all accidents occur in the home.

We face a wide variety of risks and dangers every day of our lives. But they don't paralyze us. We educate ourselves about the risks, do what we can to minimize them, and go on about our lives.

Every day we make choices that affect our safety. We decide how fast to drive, how high to climb, how far out to swim. We measure the relative risk of one action over another. We decide whether the benefit of the action is worth the risk involved in undertaking it.

Well, the risks and dangers from taking natural estrogen replacement are far less than the risks and dangers from any of the activities mentioned above. And the benefits far exceed the benefits of those activities.

Why haven't I heard any of this before?

Chapter 16

People would rather discuss religion or politics.

Female hormones… menopause… vaginal dryness… How comfortable do you feel discussing these things? Most women feel uncomfortable discussing anything connected with sex. People don't have trouble discussing thyroid (a hormone!) or insulin (another hormone!), but mention estrogen… People blush and the conversation fades to a halt. And thus the subject has remained somewhat mysterious. Folk explanations, old wives tales and home remedies have been allowed to take the place of scientific facts.

We don't want people to think we are old.

Despite the vast number of baby-boomers in our population, our society is still very youth-oriented. We don't like calling attention to our age by discussing things that make us sound old. (And what sounds older than menopause?) So we avoid discussing the very important changes taking place in our bodies. We don't want acquaintances to know we are "that old," as it might affect how they treat us socially or professionally. Nor do we seek advice on such matters from

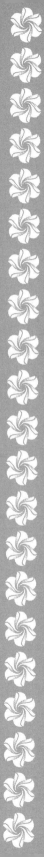

older friends, as we don't want to offend them by implying they might be old enough to have answers!

What was there to know?

Up until about 20-25 years ago, scientific information about hormones was pretty much limited to the scientific community—and they didn't know all that much. There had been little or no research on the chemical changes that took place in women's bodies when their ovaries quit producing hormones. There were no accurate tests to measure hormone levels in the blood stream.

What little we did hear or read about estrogen was related to the early birth control pills and had nothing at all to do with estrogen replacement therapy, but many people confused the issues. When birth control pills came onto the market, we learned that these pills contained artificial female hormones. Then we discovered that a very small percentage of women using "the pill" were experiencing serious side effects. Two and two were immediately added up to five: hormones were unnatural, and they might harm you.

Menopause, on the other hand, was still considered a natural state of affairs. Nobody had a clue about estrogen deficiency, and the harm it could do.

When natural estrogen finally came onto the scene to reduce the annoying symptoms of menopause, some physicians were cautious. They under-prescribed, "just to be on the safe side." And when women complained that their treatment wasn't doing

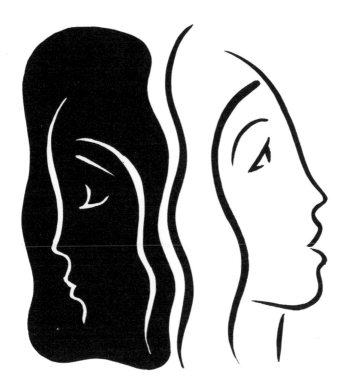

any good, the already skeptical physicians were easily convinced to discontinue it.

Even worse, some misguided gurus of "eternal youth" over-prescribed the new hormones. They apparently thought if a little was good, more must be better. And their patients began manifesting alarming side-effects brought on by over-dosage of unbuffered estrogen.

Remember—until recently, there was no useful way to measure hormone levels to guide treatment.

And in those early days of hormone replacement therapy, nothing was known about balancing estrogen with progesterone to prevent endometrial cancer. What was becoming well-known was the disturbing fact that people who took estrogen had a higher rate of cancer in the uterine lining.

All of these circumstances led to a number of legitimate questions about the safety and usefulness of hormones—questions which linger in many minds even now, many years later.

"Have things really changed?"

Yes! Extensive research has been done on the chemical changes that occur when a woman's ovaries stop producing hormones—and on the short- and long-term effects of those chemical changes. Very specific blood tests have been developed to measure the amount of hormones circulating within a woman's body. And estrogen replacement therapy for women now includes progesterone replacement therapy, which protects the lining of the uterus from the stimulating effects of the estrogen.

There is an enormous amount of knowledge on the subject of estrogen deficiency and estrogen replacement therapy. But many women remain too self-conscious, too age-conscious, or too unconsciously fearful to seek out the information. Unfortunately, this is one instance where what you don't know can hurt you.

86

Your future... your choice.

Chapter 17

Throughout this book, we have been discussing the importance of treating estrogen deficiency with estrogen replacement therapy. What we are really talking about is the quality of your life.

Life has two major dimensions. One measures the length of your life in hours, days, months and years. A perhaps more important dimension measures the quality of those hours.

As individuals, each of us must evaluate the quality of our own lives. No one else in the world can experience the ups and downs of how we feel. No one else can truly feel our pain or pleasure. That's what makes it so easy for others to make light of what we say we are feeling. After all, if they're not hurting, they can't imagine why we should be.

While sometimes aggravating, this inability of others to understand what we are experiencing is not a bad thing. It merely forces us to assume a certain amount of responsibility for the quality of our own lives. We only have a finite number of days on this planet. It's up to us to continually assess our options and determine the best way to live out those days.

This concept of individual choice certainly applies to your decision regarding estrogen replacement therapy. Estrogen deficiency can have a significant impact upon the quality of your life. We've talked a lot about some of the consequences, but there are still others you may not be aware of. Here's a partial list:

- **bone loss (osteoporosis)**
- **increased plaque formation in the arteries**
- **up to a 40% increase in the incidence of Alzheimer's Disease**
- **decreased contact lens comfort**
- **decreased short-term memory**
- **increased urinary tract infections**
- **carpal tunnel syndrome**
- **insomnia**
- **hot flashes**
- **anxiety attacks**
- **depression (including postpartum depression, or "baby blues")**
- **premenstrual depression and mood changes**
- **irritability**
- **decreased energy levels**
- **poor concentration**

- **decreased vitality**
- **poor sex life**
- **mood swings**
- **decreased collagen content in the skin**
- **increased sweating, especially "night sweats"**
- **decreased ability to take part in daily activities**
- **loss of work or reduction in social life due to increase in health-related problems**
- **decreased self-control**
- **decreased sense of well-being**
- **increased feeling of social isolation**
- **increased fibromyalgia (muscular pain)**
- **increased joint pain**

… And the list goes on.

It's a long list. And it's really up to you whether or not you choose to risk having those things impact upon the quality of your life. Sure—some women get lucky and never experience any of those problems. Other women may experience a couple of them, or several of them, or darn near all of them. Untreated estrogen deficiency is like putting your life on the line and rolling the dice.

You can't assure yourself of the outcome based upon the experiences of someone else. Perhaps they were one of the lucky ones; perhaps not. They can advise us, but that advice only relates to what they have felt. Their luck isn't your luck, and their willingness to tolerate pain and discomfort is no indicator of your need to do so.

Scientific evidence and medical statistics should be your guide. And the mountain of research documentation now available on estrogen deficiency says estrogen replacement therapy can significantly improve the quality—and length—of your life.

"Aren't there other things I can do to improve the quality of my life?"

Yes, indeed! I said at the outset that this book was neither a textbook nor an encyclopedia. While this book has dealt exclusively with the subjects of hormone deficiency, and hormone replacement therapy, that doesn't mean there aren't other areas that impact upon the quality of your life. Estrogen replacement is not the only step you can take to maintain your health, improve your outlook on life, reduce your stress level and sharpen your mental skills. Three major things come immediately to mind:

1 If you smoke, stop.

Breaking this habit will improve your attitude (you'll be less irritable, breathe easier, cough less frequently). It will help your bones stay stronger, improve your circulation and oxygenation, and decrease your risk of contracting any number of a long list of smoking-related diseases.

Best advice: If you smoke, stop now.

However, stopping smoking will not correct estrogen deficiency. Only estrogen replacement therapy can do that.

2 Exercise.

Exercise is terrific for your physical and mental conditioning. It helps strengthen your bones and improves your circulation. It also releases endorphins (the body's natural pain-relieving chemicals) into your system that improve your mood. But each person differs in their tolerance for physical exercise, so you may need advice on how much and what type of exercise is best for you.

However, exercise does not correct the problem of estrogen deficiency. Only estrogen replacement can do that.

3 Adopt a healthy diet.

A good diet is another basic foundation of good health. Learn all you can about what constitutes a good diet, and make changes in your eating habits accordingly.

But remember: good nutrition does not correct estrogen deficiency. Only estrogen replacement can do that.

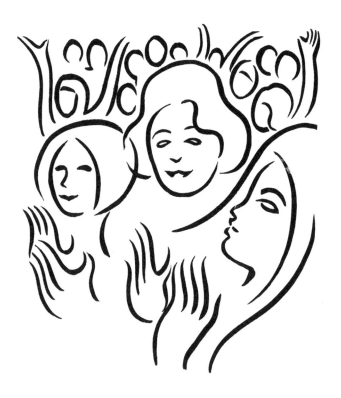

"You keep coming back to estrogen replacement therapy."

That's because estrogen deficiency is a preventable, highly treatable condition—but one that can only be treated by replacing at least minimal amounts of your body's natural supply of estrogen.

This book has presented you with a lot of information about the dangers of estrogen deficiency, and the benefits of estrogen replacement therapy. Most of all, it has presented you with a choice.

Women once had no options. If they survived their child-bearing years, they were faced with the inevitable, unpleasant, and potentially deadly consequences of estrogen deficiency. They had no choice in the matter.

You do. You can correct your estrogen deficiency and continue leading a rational, healthy, active life. Or you can "suffer through it" like generations of women have done before you and risk your cardio-vascular health, your bone structure, and your mental and emotional stability. It's your choice.

You have taken the first step by reading this book and becoming better informed. The next step is to make an appointment with your health care professional. Bring along this book for reference, and a list of any questions you still have. Together, you can discuss your alternatives and decide what is best in your individual situation.

If you are not comfortable with your doctor's recommendations, you also have the choice of consulting another doctor for a second opinion. Don't feel shy about asking for a second opinion—it's important for you to feel right about your health care decisions.

It's your future... and your choice.

References

Hundreds of references in the current scientific literature were studied in researching information for this book. A few of these references are listed here as an aid to those who wish to do further independent study. They are listed in groups by subject. Nearly all authors are physicians and nearly all articles are from major, peer-reviewed journals.

SUBJECT: BREAST CANCER

FITZGERALD, CHERYL T., *et al*: Review: Hormone replacement therapy and malignancy. British Journal of Obstetrics and Gynecology May 1993; Vol. 100, pp. 408-410. (35 references)

> *Conclusion*: "The fears over the increased incidence of gynecological and breast malignancies associated with oestrogen replacement therapy are not justified, and women should not be denied treatment on those grounds."

SMELLIE, W. JAMES B. & THOMAS, J. MEIRION: Hormone replacement therapy and breast cancer. British Journal of Obstetrics and Gynecology May 1993; Vol. 100, pp. 404-407. (50 references)

> *Conclusion*: "Sufficient data now exist to support the view that short term use of oestrogen replacement therapy does not have a clinically significant link with breast cancer."

COLDITZ, GRAHAM A., *et al*: Hormone replacement therapy and risk of breast cancer: Results from epidimiologic studies. American Journal of Obstetrics and Gynecology 1993; Vol. 168, pp 1473-80. (Meta-analysis, 24 references)

> *Conclusion*: "Although these results exclude a large effect of hormone therapy on risk of breast cancer, we are unable to rule out some risk associated with current or long term use estrogen use."

ZUMOFF, B.: Review: Biological and endocrinological insights into the possible breast cancer risk from menopausal estrogen replacement therapy. Steroids May 1993; Vol. 58, pp 196-204. (141 references)

> Conclusion: "At present, the majority of investigators agree that short-term or medium-term therapy (less than 10 years) poses no measurable risk; some, but not all, investigators feel that there is a modest risk with long-term therapy (more than 15 years). Even this semi-consensus is clouded by the startling and clear-cut finding of the largest ever epidemiological study, the Nurses Surveillance Study, that a small increase in risk with estrogen therapy occurred only in women who also ingested alcohol, itself a known risk factor for breast cancer; women who did not ingest alcohol were at no increased risk."

GAMBRELL, R. DON, JR.: Estrogen Replacement Therapy and Breast Cancer Risk, A New Look at the Data. The Female Patient April 1993; Vol. 18, pp 50-62. (43 references)

> Conclusion: "After presenting a thorough review of the data, this paper concludes that exogenous estrogen does not contribute to breast cancer risk and furthermore that adding progestogens to the regimen may actually reduce the risk."

NACHTIGALL, LILA E., & NACHTIGALL, MARGARET J.: Review: Hormone Replacement Therapy. Current Opinion in Obstetrics and Gynecology December 1992; Vol. 4, pp 907-913. (68 references)

> Conclusion: "It is clear that in the average, healthy woman, low-dose estrogen replacement for less than 10 years does not increase the risk of breast cancer."

NACHTIGALL, MARGARET J., et al: Incidence of Breast Cancer in a 22-Year Study of Women Receiving Estrogen-Progestin Replacement Therapy. Obstetrics and Gynecology November 1992; Vol. 80, pp 827-30. (Original research)

> Conclusion: "These data suggest that the 22-year administration of estrogen-progestin hormone replacement

therapy did not increase the incidence of breast cancer in a small group of continuously hospitalized post-menopausal women."

Ed. note: *168 women were continuously observed in a hospital setting for* **22 years**. *Those who received hormone replacement therapy had* **no** *breast cancers. However, 11.5 % of those who had* **never** *taken hormone replacement therapy developed breast cancer (the same incidence as expected in the U. S. general population).*

HENRICH, JANET B.: Review: The Postmenopausal Estrogen/Breast Cancer Controversy. Journal of the American Medical Association October 1992; Vol 268, pp 1900-1902. (35 references)

Conclusion: "These findings do not support an overall increased risk of breast cancer in women who ever used postmenopausal estrogens or a conclusive or consistent effect across other measures of use. Cross-national differences in estrogen use and inequalities in breast cancer detection between estrogen users and nonusers may account for the increased risk estimates reported in some studies."

STRICKLAND, DANIEL M., et al: The Relationship Between Breast Cancer Survival and Prior Postmenopausal Estrogen Use. Obstetrics and Gynecology September 1992; Vol. 80, pp 400-404. (38 references)

Conclusion: "We conclude that prior postmenopausal estrogen replacement therapy does not compromise survival in women who subsequently develop carcinoma of the breast."

KHOO, SOO KEAT & CHICK, PAMELA: Sex steroid hormones and breast cancer: is there a link with oral contraceptives and hormone replacement therapy? The Medical Journal of Australia January 1992; Vol. 156, pp 124-132. (103 references)

Conclusion: "The review revealed good evidence that use of sex steroid hormones had no significant effect on the risk of breast cancer, whether given for contraception or hormone replacement."

WILE, ALAN G. & DiSAIA, PHILIP J.: Hormones and Breast Cancer. The American Journal of Surgery April 1989; Vol. 157, pp 438-442. (39 references)

Conclusion: "In conclusion, there is no substantial evidence that there is any association between high levels of female hormones, whether endogenous or exogenous, with increased risk of development of breast cancer or exacerbation of preexisting breast cancer."

SUBJECT: CARDIOVASCULAR DISEASE

WENGER, NANETTE K., et al: Cardiovascular Health and Disease in Women. The New England Journal of Medicine July 1993; Vol. 329, pp. 247-256. (138 references)

Conclusion: "Observational studies suggest a reduction of approximately 50 percent in the risk of coronary heart disease among healthy postmenopausal women taking oral estrogen, with an even more substantial benefit among women with documented coronary heart disease. Hypertension, diabetes, and a history of stroke are not contraindications to estrogen therapy."

WREN, BARRY G.: The effect of oestrogen on the female cardiovascular system. The Medical Journal of Australia August 1992; Vol. 157, pp. 204-208. (103 references)

Conclusion: "The consensus of the published data is that oestrogen conveys a highly protective effect on the cardiovascular system of postmenopausal women. There will be a reduction of up to 50% in myocardial infarction and stroke, a reduction in the incidence of hypertension and an improvement in blood flow. Some of the data suggest that even for women who have suffered from an infarct, their long-term survival is enhanced by oestrogen therapy."

SOMA, MAURIZIO R., PHD, et al: The Lowering of Lipoprotein(a) Induced by Estrogen Plus Progesterone

Replacement Therapy in Postmenopausal Women. Archives of Internal Medicine June 1993; Vol. 153, pp. 1462-1468. (Original investigation)

> *Conclusion*: "The results suggest that in estrogen plus progesterone-treated postmenopausal women, the lipid profile is improved not only by lowering low-density lipoprotein cholesterol levels and raising high-density lipoprotein levels, but also lowering plasma Lp(a) concentrations."

NABLUSI, AZMI A., *et al*: Association of Hormone-Replacement Therapy with Various Cardiovascular Risk Factors in Postmenopausal Women. The New England Journal of Medicine April 1993; Vol. 328, pp. 1069-75. (50 references)

> *Conclusion*: "Hormone-replacement therapy appears to be associated with a favorable physiologic profile, which probably mediates its protective effects on cardiovascular disease. The use of estrogen combined with progestin appears to be associated with a better profile than the use of estrogen alone."

MARTIN, KATHRYN A. & FREEMAN, MASON W.: Editorial: Postmenopausal Hormone-Replacement Therapy. The New England Journal of Medicine April 1993; Vol. 328, pp. 1115-17. (Editorial)

> *Conclusion*: "While we await further information from prospective, clinical trials such as the Women's Health Initiative (sponsored by the National Institutes of Health), what are women and their physicians to do? On the basis of the available evidence, we recommend that all postmenopausal women be considered candidates for hormone-replacement therapy and be educated about its risks and benefits."

FALKEBORN, MARGARETA, *et al*: The risk of acute myocardial infarction after oestrogen and oestrogen-progestogen replacement. British Journal of Obstetrics and Gynecology October 1992; Vol. 99, pp. 821-828. (Original investigation)

> *Conclusion*: "Hormonal replacement therapy with oestrogens alone, and maybe also when cyclically combined

with progestogens, can reduce the risk of acute myocardial infarction."

FALKEBORN, MARGARETA, et al: Hormone Replacement Therapy and the Risk of Stroke. Follow-up of a Population-Based Cohort in Sweden. Archives of Internal Medicine May 1993; Vol.153, pp. 1201-1209. (Original investigation)

Conclusion: "Hormone replacement therapy with potent estrogens alone or cyclically combined with progestins can, particularly when started shortly after menopause, reduce the risk of stroke."

LINDENSTROM, EWA, et al: Lifestyle Factors and Risk of Cerebrovascular Disease in Women. The Copenhagen City Heart Study. Stroke October 1993; Vol. 24, pp. 1468-1472. (Original investigation)

Conclusion: "In postmenopausal women, there was a statistically significant interaction between smoking and hormone replacement therapy. Smokers receiving this therapy had a 28% lower risk of cerebrovascular disease than smokers not receiving it."

SUBJECT: ENDOMETRIAL CANCER PREVENTION WITH PROGESTERONE

NYHOLMM, HENRIK CHRISTIAN JUUL, et al: Endometrial Cancer in Postmenopausal Women with and without Previous Estrogen Replacement Treatment: Comparison of Clinical and Histopathological Characteristics. Gynecologic Oncology 1993; Vol. 49, pp. 229-235. (Original investigation)

Conclusion: "Our findings support the theory that endometrial cancer of estrogen users may be less aggressive than cancer of nonusers."

LUCIANO, ANTHONY A., et al: Evaluation of Low-Dose Estrogen and Progestin Therapy in Postmenopausal Women: A Double-Blind, Prospective Study of Sequential Versus Continuous Therapy. The Journal of Reproductive Medicine March 1993; Vol. 38, pp. 207-214. (Original investigation)

Conclusion: Their data showed sequential therapy reduced but did not eliminate endometrial proliferation but "continuous use of MPA at either the 2.5 or 5.0 mg daily dose, induces amenorrhea within 4-6 months and results in consistent endometrial atrophy."

MACLENNAN, ALASTAIR H., *et al*: Continuous low-dose oestrogen and progestogen hormone replacement therapy: a randomized trial. The Medical Journal of Australia July 1993; Vol. 159, pp. 102-106. (Original investigation)

Conclusion: "These low-dose continuous estrogen and progestogen regimens appear an appropriate option for the postmenopausal woman wishing to eliminate withdrawal bleeding and reduce both hormonal side effects and menopausal symptoms."

LOBO, ROGERIO A.: The Role of Progestins in Hormone Replacement Therapy. American Journal of Obstetrics and Gynecology June 1992; Vol.166, pp. 1997-2004. (55 references)

Conclusion: "Progestins are used to prevent endometrial hyperplasia and carcinoma but should not be prescribed for women who have had hysterectomies. Doses that decrease mitotic activity are sufficient."; "...it is advisable to use sufficient estrogen and minimum progestin."; "...it is my view that progestins should be administered sequentially with the use of a lower dose (2.5 to 5 mg of MPA, 1 mg of NET) for only 10 days."

GAMBRELL, R. DON, JR.: Pathophysiology and Epidemiology of Endometrial Cancer. Treatment of the Postmenopausal Woman: Basic and Clinical Aspects, edited by Rogerio A. Lobo, Raven Press, Ltd., New York, 1994.

Conclusion: "With cyclic sequential addition of progestogens, the duration of progestogens should be for at least 12 to 14 days each month.";

"... norethindrone or norethindrone acetate... 1 to 2.5 mg... [or] 10 mg MPA... will fully protect the endometrium."

MOYER, DEAN L., *et al*: Prevention of endometrial hyperplasia by progesterone during long-term estradiol replacement: influence of bleeding pattern and secretory changes. Fertility and Sterility May 1993; Vol. 59, pp. 992-7. (Original investigation)

> Conclusion: "Consistent reduction in mitosis rates in glandular epithelium was found after 9 or more days of (progestogen) administration in each cycle.";
>
> "Induction of withdrawal bleeding and endometrial secretory transformation, which require larger doses of progesterone, do not provide additional benefit for prevention of hyperplasia."

GAMBRELL, R. DON, JR.: Progestogens and Postmenopausal Women. The Female Patient April 1992; Vol. 17, pp. 33-52. (31 references)

> Conclusion: "Adding progestogens to postmenopausal estrogen replacement therapy is a well-accepted means of reducing the risk of estrogen-induced endometrial cancer.";
>
> "Side effects from added progestogens may be severe in a small percentage of women. However, by adding a mild diuretic, changing the type, dosage, or route of administration, usually a progestogen can be found for symptom-free (hormone replacement therapy)."

SUBJECT: ESTROGEN BLOOD LEVELS

(See references listed under other subjects which also discuss blood estrogen levels.)

SPEROFF, LEON: Clinical Technique: The Perimenopausal Patient. OB/GYN Clinical Alert December 1993; pp. 62-64. (Opinion)

> Conclusion: Blood estrogen levels are an important tool in managing estrogen replacement therapy. His lab uses a range of 40-150 pg/mL. Since FSH is influenced by other factors it is not a useful indicator of estrogen levels.

DELIGNIERES, BRUNO AND MOYER, DEAN L.: Influence of Sex Hormones on Hyperplasia/Carcinoma Risks. Treatment of the Postmenopausal Woman: Basic and Clinical Aspects, edited by Rogerio Logo, Raven Press, Ltd., New York 1994.

> *Conclusion*: "The suitable estradiol plasma level is between 50 and 150 pg/mL during treatment."

SUBJECT: OSTEOPOROSIS

NOTELOVITZ, MORRIS: Osteoporosis: screening, prevention, and management. Fertility and Sterility April 1993; Vol. 59, pp. 707-25. (110 references)

> *Conclusion*: "Primary care physicians, especially gynecologists, can play a pivotal role by (1) identifying women with higher risks for osteoporosis at earlier ages; (2) stressing the importance of developing maximal bone mass before menopause; and (3) developing individualized patient prescriptions for bone mass determinants under personal control: exercise, nutrition (e.g., calcium and vitamin D), life-style, and hormone replacement therapy."

REGINSTER, J.Y., *et al*: Minimal levels of serum estradiol prevent postmenopausal bone loss. Calcif. Tissue Int. November 1992; Vol. 51, pp. 340-3. (Original investigation)

> *Conclusion*: "We suggest that oral or percutaneous estrogen replacement therapy should induce a minimal value of 60 pg/ml to prevent postmenopausal bone loss."

FULEIHAN, GHADA EL-HAJJ, *et al*: Effect of Sequential and Daily Continuous Hormone Replacement Therapy on Indexes of Mineral Metabolism. Archives of Internal Medicine September 1992; Vol. 152, pp. 1904-1909. (Original investigation)

> *Conclusion*: "The daily continuous estrogen-progesterone regimens are as efficacious as sequential hormone therapy in decreasing indexes of bone turnover and stabilizing bone mineral density of the spine and proximal femur."

SAVVAS, M., *et al*: Increase in bone mass after one year of percutaneous oestradiol and testosterone implants in post-menopausal women who have previously received long-term oral oestrogens. British Journal of Obstetrics and Gynecology September 1992; Vol. 99, pp. 757-760. (Original investigation)

Conclusion: "Subcutaneous oestradiol and testosterone implants will result in an increase in bone mass even after many years of oral oestrogen replacement therapy." (Ed. note: These implants are not available in the U.S. but soon should be.)

NAESSEN, TORD, et al: Maintained bone density at advanced ages after long term treatment with low dose oestradiol implants. British Journal of Obstetrics and Gynecology May 1993; Vol. 100, pp. 454-459. (Original investigation)

Conclusion: "Continuous long term treatment with low dose oestradiol implants yielding physiological levels of serum oestradiol preserves both compact and cancellous bone and the effect seems to persist into advanced ages without any inevitable age related bone loss." (Ed. note: These implants are not yet available in the U.S. but soon should be.)

HILLNER, BRUCE E., et al: Postmenopausal Estrogens in Prevention of Osteoporosis: Benefit Virtually without Risk if Cardiovascular Effects Are Considered. The American Journal of Medicine June 1986; Vol. 80, pp. 1115-1127. (61 references)

Conclusion: "Thus, estrogen therapy provides a significant gain in quality-adjusted life expectancy... Any recommendation about postmenopausal estrogens with respect to osteoporosis that excludes their cardiovascular effects markedly underestimates the potential gain from therapy."

RAVNIKAR, VERONICA A.: Hormonal Management of Osteoporosis. Clinical Obstetrics and Gynecology December 1992; Vol. 35, pp. 913-922. (38 references)

Conclusion: "If we are to make an impact on preventive care with estrogen therapy, we should increase compliance in

our patients by clearly explaining the end-points of therapy, the dramatic consequences of osteoporosis, and the
safety of such therapy."

CONSENSUS DEVELOPMENT CONFERENCE: Prophylaxis and
Treatment of Osteoporosis. The American Journal of
Medicine January 1991; Vol. 90, pp. 107-110.

Conclusion: "Osteoporosis can be prevented. Estrogen
therapy is the drug of choice for preventing bone loss in
women after the menopause or in women with
impaired ovarian function...There is yet no evidence
that moderate physical exercise retards bone loss associated with menopause or aging. However, active exercise is considered useful in the elderly, particularly in
improving muscular function and agility and in reducing the likelihood of falls."

MOYER, DEAN L., et al: Prevention of endometrial hyperplasia by progesterone during long-term estradiol replacement: influence of bleeding pattern and secretory changes.
Fertility and Sterility May 1993; Vol. 59, pp. 992-7.
(Original investigation)

Conclusion: Treatment raised blood estradiol levels to
approximately 80 pg/mL. This level prevents bone loss.
Preferable treatment is lowest dose of estrogen and progesterone which will prevent osteoporosis and also prevent endometrial overgrowth. "The higher doses inducing
withdrawal bleeding and completely developed secretory
changes do not substantially improve safety but are likely
to increase noncompliance in majority of users."

STUDD, J., et al: The relationship between plasma estradiol
and the increase in bone density in postmenopausal women
after treatment with subcutaneous hormone implants.
American Journal of Obstetrics and Gynecology November
1990; Vol. 163, pp. 1474-9. (Original investigation)

Conclusion: Pretreatment blood levels of approximately
20 pg/mL. were increased to approximately 125 pg/mL.
"The percentage increase of vertebral bone density was
not related to age, number of years past the

menopause, pretreatment bone density, or serum testosterone levels, but a significant correlation was found between the percentage increase in bone density at the spine and the serum estradiol level."

SUBJECT: QUALITY OF LIFE

WIKLUND, INGELA, *et al*: Quality of life of postmenopausal women on a regimen of transdermal estradiol therapy: A double-blind placebo-controlled study. American Journal of Obstetrics and Gynecology March 1993; Vol. 168, pp. 824-30. (Original investigation)

> Conclusion: This study reports statistically significant improvement for those taking estrogen versus a placebo in many areas of life including: Sleep, social isolation, emotions, energy, well-being, anxiety, vitality, self-control, depression, physical symptoms, hot flashes/night sweats, thinking/ reasoning/memory, sexual problems, and sexual satisfaction.

SUBJECT: REVIEW, EXTENSIVE

SMITH, N.J. ROGER & STUDD, JOHN W.W.: Recent advances in hormone replacement therapy. British Journal of Hospital Medicine 1993; Vol. 49, pp. 799-808. (66 references)

> Conclusion: "Every postmenopausal woman should be offered the potential benefits of (hormone replacement therapy), but particularly those with heart disease, depression, and osteoporosis. These are the very patients who are often denied (hormone replacement therapy) for illogical reasons."

MARSHBURN, PAUL B. & CARR, BRUCE R.: Hormone Replacement therapy: Protection against the consequences of menopause. Postgraduate Medicine September 1992; Vol. 92, pp. 145-159. (39 references)

> Conclusion: "Most postmenopausal women are candidates for for such therapy, which has beneficial effects on serum cholesterol levels and other cardiovascular

risk factors and protects against osteoporosis, urogenital atrophy, and vasomotor symptoms. A small number of patients have specific risk factors for or contraindications to hormone replacement therapy."

HARLAP, SUSAN (MB, BS): The benefits and risks of hormone replacement therapy: An epidemiologic overview. American Journal of Obstetrics and Gynecology June 1992; Vol. 166, pp. 1986-92. (51 references)

Conclusion: "Current epidemiologic knowledge suggests that the benefits of hormone replacement therapy, with or without any progestins, strongly outweigh the risks."

GAMBRELL, R. DON, JR.: Update on Hormone Replacement Therapy. Supplement to American Family Physician November 1992; Vol. 46, pp. 87S-96S. (39 references)

Clinical opinion article which sites extensive evidence for the lack of increased breast cancer risk with hormone replacement therapy. The author asserts "All published studies have reported" that women with breast cancer survived longer if they were receiving hormone replacement therapy at the time of its diagnosis.

SESSION, DONNA R., et al: Current concepts in estrogen replacement therapy in the menopause. Fertility and Sterility February 1993; Vol. 59, pp. 277-84. (92 references)

Conclusion: "New therapeutic regimens and modes of delivery decrease risks and increase patient acceptance of hormonal replacement therapy."

ZUBIALDE, JOHN P., et al: Estimated Gains in Life Expectancy with Use of Postmenopausal Estrogen Therapy: A Decision Analysis. The Journal of Family Practice 1993; Vol. 36, pp. 271-280. (38 references)

Original epidemiological research article which concludes: "Substantial increases in life expectancy may result from postmenopausal estrogen therapy. These may be equal to or possibly greater than benefits from other well-recognized risk-reduction strategies."

SUBJECT: TESTOSTERONE

BACHMANN, GLORIA A.: Estrogen-Androgen Therapy for Sexual and Emotional Well-Being. The Female Patient July 1993; Vol. 18, pp. 15-24. (26 references)

Conclusion: Review article presents evidence for effectiveness of estrogen-androgen therapy to increase sexual desire and well-being.

YOUNG, RONALD L.: Androgens in postmenopausal therapy? Menopause Management May 1993; pp. 21-24. (18 references)

Conclusion: Review article cites evidence for the safety and effectiveness of estrogen-androgen therapy for improvement of libido and well-being.

SUBJECT: VENOUS THROMBOSIS

LOBO, ROGERIO A.: Editorial: Estrogen and the Risk of Coagulopathy. The American Journal of Medicine March 1992; Vol. 92, pp. 283-5. (21 references)

Conclusion: "Practitioners should not be concerned about modest 'replacement' doses of estrogen in terms of the risk of coagulopathy. Clearly, synthetic estrogens (Ed. note: birth control pills) should be avoided unless the doses are extremely low...On the basis of current information, postmenopausal estrogen therapy is of value and should be prescribed without fear."

DEVOR, MICHELLE, et al: Estrogen Replacement Therapy and the Risk of Venous Thrombosis. The American Journal of Medicine March 1992; Vol. 92, pp. 275-282. (50 references)

Conclusion: "This case-control study of older women, unselected for other thrombotic risk factors, does not support the commonly held assumption that replacement estrogen increases the risk of venous thrombosis."

Publisher's Cataloging in Publication
(Prepared by Quality Books, Inc.)

Sevener, M.D., C. Alan.
  It's Okay to Take Estrogen: In fact estrogen may be
your best friend for life / C. Alan Sevener, M.D.
p. cm.
Includes bibliographical references.
ISBN 0-9642282-9-7

  1. Estrogen—Therapeutic use. 2. Menopause—
Hormone therapy. I. Title

RG186.S48 1995   618.1'75'061
                                      QBI94-2197

Thanks to Marsha Anderson, Editor.
C.A.S.

111

If you are unable to find additional copies of this book at your local bookstore please ask them to order them for you. Or you may order from Eclectic Publishing, Inc.

Mail your order payable to:
E.P.I.—It's Okay Book
P.O. Box 28340
Fresno, CA 93729-8340

Or you may call or fax your order:
1-209-434-3549
Fax 1-209-434-0448

Include shipping fee of $3.00 for first book and $1.00 for each additional book sent in a single order to the same address. Visa and Mastercard credit card orders must include card number and expiration date. Orders to California addresses must include 7.85% state sales tax ($1.17 per book).

_____ copies It's Okay to Take Estrogen @ $14.95 **COST $**_____

(CA only) TAX $_____

SHIPPING $_____

TOTAL $_____

❑ VISA ❑ MasterCard

Credit Card # _____

Exp. Date_____

Signature_____

Ship to:_____
      NAME

      ADDRESS

      CITY   STATE   ZIP

      PHONE   FAX

Eclectic Publishing welcomes your comments and suggestions. Feel free to contact us at any time. We value your opinion.

(Photocopy this form for placing orders by mail or fax.)